Ancient Wisdom for Fitness and Nutrition

Applying Tradition to Modern Life

Table of Contents

Chapter 1. Introduction

Embrace the past to enhance your present with our Special Report, "Ancient Wisdom for Fitness and Nutrition: Applying Tradition to Modern Life." Filled with rousing anecdotes, cutting-edge research findings, and engaging narratives, this literature brilliantly links time-honored traditional practices to contemporary wellness techniques. As far removed from technical verbosity as can be, this report teems instead with rejuvenating and exciting insights into fitness and nutrition that our ancestors aced, and we seem to have overlooked. Unveil the secrets of our forebears, rediscover the power of nature and tradition, and reshape your wellness journey! An enticing fusion of the old and the new awaits your exploration – a purchase that will surely prove to be an investment in health and happiness.

Chapter 2. Ancient Roots of Wellness: An Introductory Glimpse

History is replete with instances of ancient societies thriving and excelling in physical prowess and dietary wisdom. Their mastery, a perfect blend of instinct, experience, and ingenuity, resonates powerfully even in our hyper-modern era. This wellness prowess, embodied in food choices, physical activities, and even spiritual routines, offers valuable insights into our present day attempts at crafting healthier lifestyles.

2.1. The Historicity of Fitness

Ancient civilizations, in their encounters with the conundrum of survival and progress, found fitness not just necessary but invaluable. Societies such as the ancient Greeks, Romans, and Egyptians incorporated physical exercise as integral parts of their daily routines and societal constructs.

In ancient Greece, for instance, the concept of a healthy mind in a healthy body reigned supreme. Gymnasiums weren't just spaces for physical exercise; they were also hubs of intellectual discourse, places where the physical and the intellectual were nurtured together. Training was comprehensive, encompassing a variety of activities that encouraged both strength and agility.

The Romans, greatly influenced by the Greeks, implemented similar fitness orientations. They established bath houses interspersed with gymnasiums where citizens engaged in exercise and social interaction alike. Acknowledging physical fitness as a determinant of a good soldier, martial training was extensive.

The civilization of the Nile, ancient Egypt, also offers fascinating fitness anecdotes. Recorded on temple walls are tales of marathons and swimming contests, suggesting an ingrained culture of physical competition.

This is not all. Far from the Mediterranean, the Shaolin monks in China developed Kung Fu not just as a martial art, but as a blend of fitness and spiritual discipline. Traditional tribal African communities too had intricate dances which simultaneously served as fun, community-building, and physically engaging exercise.

2.2. The Wisdom in Nutrition

Paralleling their understanding of physical fitness, ancient societies were surprisingly insightful when it came to nutrition. Our ancestors, through observation and experience, seemed to possess an intuitive grasp of dietary wisdom.

The longevity of the Okinawans in Japan is often attributed to their traditional diet, whole and rich in fiber. The Inuit people thrived in the Arctic, despite it being an ostensibly inhospitable environment, due to a diet rich in omega-3 fatty acids found in fish and other marine life.

In ancient India, the Ayurvedic system of medicine, believed to be at least three millennia old, identifies ideal dietary practices based on individual constitutions, made up of the three Doshas: Vata, Pitta and Kapha. Ayurveda encourages the consumption of seasonal and regional foods, establishing a dietary rhythm closely in sync with nature.

Even the ancient Greeks understood the link between food and health. Hippocrates, widely considered the father of medicine, famously said, "Let food be thy medicine, and medicine be thy food," highlighting the pivotal role diet plays in health and well-being.

2.3. The Power of Rituals

Ancient practices were not restricted to the realm of fitness and nutrition alone. Rituals and traditions, emanating from a deep connection with nature and spirituality, were also significant facets of their lifestyle. This is visible in the Inuits' respect for the animals they hunted, traditional African gratitude rituals around harvest time, or Hindu practices of beginning every day with sunrise yoga and meditation.

These rituals were not just for the sake of spirituality; many had undeniable health benefits. Traditional Chinese practices like acupuncture and Tai Chi, or Indian yoga and meditation, are widely recognized today for their therapeutic benefits. Even the act of gathering around a fire, a practice central to many ancient cultures, has been linked to benefits like reduced blood pressure and increased social bonds.

How these practices affect us may not always be clear, but the fact that they work is irrefutable. Science is only starting to catch up, and every finding seems to endorse the adage - there is wisdom in tradition.

As we unearth the relics of ancient fitness and nutrition, we must recognize the value of these practices, not just in their historical context, but as conduits to enhance our understanding of contemporary wellness techniques. In this wisdom of the ages lies the potential to shape our lifestyle, perfect our nutritional choices and redefine our standards of fitness and health for the better.

Our ancestors may not have had scientific terminology and a methodical approach to articulate their wisdom, but their empirical knowledge remains an invaluable trove, oftentimes richer and deeper than our modern understanding. As we grapple with the consequences of our fast-paced, technology-driven lifestyles, perhaps we should turn back to the keepers of the old ways. And in their wisdom, find our way back to the roots of wellness.

Chapter 3. Deciphering the Nutritional Patterns of Our Ancestors

Our ancestors, devoid of modern conveniences and technology, relied heavily on their understanding of nature and their bodies to survive and thrive. As we venture through this exploration of traditional nutritional patterns, we should bear in mind that these ancestral diets were geographically and culturally specific. Hence comparisons and not exact matches will provide us with the most practical applications for our current lifestyles.

3.1. The Paleolithic Diet

Think back to a time before agriculture was introduced, when humans were hunter-gatherers. This is the era of the Paleolithic or Stone Age diet. The diet was incredibly diverse and depended substantially on the location and season. It primarily comprised wild game, seasonal fruits, nuts, and seeds, berries, fish, and occasionally honey. The absence of dairy, grains, or added sugars is a distinguishing feature. This diet provided a balanced ratio of macronutrients and was replete with fiber, vitamins, and minerals, but low in sodium. However, the Paleolithic era had its seasons of scarcity, pressing man to go long hours, even days, fasting or surviving on a minimal diet.

3.2. The Neolithic Revolution and Its Impact on Diet

With the advent of the Neolithic period and the invention of agriculture, human diet underwent a significant shift. Grains and cereals, dairy products, and legumes—fare previously unavailable or scarce—became cornerstones of the human diet. Domesticated animals supplemented wild game. Fermented beverages, including beer and wine, also appeared during this era. Grain-based foods might have increased the carbohydrate intake, but they were fat and protein-rich, thanks to the whole grains and method of preparation, quite distinct from today's processed, high-carb, low-fiber counterparts.

3.3. Traditional Asian and Mediterranean Diets

The traditional Asian and Mediterranean diets offer a geographical move from our Paleolithic and Neolithic ancestors. The Asian diet typically centers on rice, noodles, and various soy products, supplemented with fish, seafood, and a vast assortment of colourful vegetables and fruits. Diversity, balance, and moderation characterize this dietary pattern.

The Mediterranean diet, drawing from various European cultures, centres around olive oil, fresh fruits and vegetables, whole grains, nuts, legumes, dairy (mainly cheese and yoghurt), and wine in moderation. Intake of red meat is limited in a Mediterranean diet. Both these diets emphasize plant-based, whole food diets rich in monosaturated fats, omega-3 fatty acids and antioxidants, which are linked to lower risks of heart disease and better overall health.

3.4. Indigenous American Diets

The diet of the Indigenous Americans was equally dependent on locally available flora and fauna. Corn, beans, squash, peppers, potatoes, tomatoes, and turkeys are only some of the food items that emerged from these groups. The indigenous peoples had remarkable techniques for preparing food like nixtamalization, a process to treat maize with alkali, reducing mycotoxin count and improving protein bioavailability and niacin content.

3.5. Food, A Social Phenomenon

Understanding the social context of food could hold critical insights into the way our ancestors ate. Eating has always been a communal exercise. Sharing food bolstered community ties and provided a sense of security and belonging - critical for survival in harsh conditions. In contrast, modern life lends itself to solitary and hurried consumption of nutritionally jeopardized meals.

3.6. Fasting and Feasting

Seasons of feast and famine punctuated the eating patterns of our ancestors. Bioavailability of food was subject to seasonal availability, fostering a cycle of fasting and feasting. Modern derivative of these practices is seen in the advent of intermittent fasting, a nutrition approach to manage weight and improve health markers.

3.7. Conclusion: Lessons from the Ancestors

Gleaning from the dietary patterns of the past, several key takeaways apply to modern nutrition. Food diversity and moderation stood out as a consistent theme through varying cultures and periods. The intake of whole, unprocessed foods rich in vitamins, minerals, and fiber was a staple. The value of community and mindful eating, along with understanding the body's need for balance, incorporating seasons of abundance and scarcity, rings true even today.

Going forward, let us use this understanding to inform our nutritional choices. Let's respect that our bodies have evolved over millions of years and in specific environments and lineages. Our diet should echo this evolution and environmental adaptation, emphasizing whole, nutrient-dense foods, and aligned, when practical, with our unique ancestries.

Chapter 4. Physical Culture in Ancient Civilizations: How they Moved

Our understanding of physical fitness traces roots far beyond the concept of modern gyms and high-tech equipment. Today, we delve into the depths of ancient civilizations' fitness cultures, with Greece, India, China, and Egypt at the helm, to gain insights into how they maneuvered their lives physically.

4.1. Ancient Greece: The Birthplace of Gymnasia

The Greeks laid the groundwork for many modern fitness concepts. They believed that a strong body signified a strong mind ("mens sana in corpore sano"), fostering the establishment of gymnasia - places for physical training, intellectual growth, and social interaction.

Most famous were the Olympic Games, from 776 BC, where athletes competed in various physical disciplines like wrestling, boxing, and chariot racing. Athenians, including philosopher Socrates, appreciated fitness, considering it a civic duty to remain physically active. Moreover, their exercise regimen included gymnastics, dancing, wrestling, and running- exercises we still enjoy today.

The Greeks also invented the 'halteres' (akin to dumbbells today) and 'diskos' (similar to discus). These tools offered strength and coordination training, indicating that the Greeks understood the importance of progressive resistance exercise for strength and health centuries ago.

4.2. Fitness in Ancient India: Yoga and Kalaripayattu

Centuries ago, in the mystic lands of India, physical fitness was intertwined with spirituality. Yoga, a discipline dating back to 3000 BC, linking breath control, meditation, and bodily postures, was practiced widely for spiritual enlightenment and physical prowess. In essence, these techniques embody resistance training, flexibility exercises, and cardio, eerily similar to some aspects of fitness training we champion today.

Furthermore, Kalaripayattu, one of the world's oldest martial arts, was developed here. This practice focused on flexibility, agility, overall body strength, and mental acuity. Much of their combat and movement system involved body-weight movements and floor-based exercises eerily similar to what we now label as functional or primal movement.

4.3. Chinese Health Culture: Qi Gong and Martial Arts

Appreciating the reciprocal relationship between mind and body, Chinese fitness culture involved harnessing energy, or 'Qi,' through various methods. Qi Gong, a collection of movements, postures, and controlled breathing techniques dating back to 2500 BC, was inherently therapeutic, investing in internal healing and strength.

Martial arts, particularly Tai Chi and Kung Fu, were popular for physical strength and self-defense. Interestingly, these martial arts included movements that fostered flexibility, strength, and cardiovascular health, analogous to modern high-intensity interval training (HIIT).

Chinese fitness traditions were widely holistic. They acknowledged the interplay between diet, movement, and mental health centuries earlier than western medicine, truly pioneers of holistic wellness.

4.4. Egypt: Hard Labor and Dance

In Ancient Egypt, physical fitness revolved mainly around labor-intensive tasks, including building colossal structures like pyramids and palaces. Such intense manual labor necessitated sound physical endurance and strength, reinforcing exercise's importance in their daily life.

Interestingly, dance held social and religious significance, embodying vigorous movements that promoted strength, agility, and aerobic conditioning. From tomb paintings and historical records, we gather that dance was central to celebrations, religious rites, and even physical therapy, pointing towards a cultural appreciation for movement and fitness.

Looking at these cultures lets us unravel the rich tapestry of traditional fitness. While our contexts and tools have changed, the fundamental principles of movement and physical fitness echo through the millenniums. The cross-cultural emphasis on regular exercise for physical health, mental clarity, and spiritual growth remains as vital today as it was in antiquity.

Understanding how our ancestors moved has significant implications for contemporary society, entrenched in sedentary lifestyles and virtual realities. This exploration reminds us of the fundamental human need for movement to maintain optimal health, a principle that predates most of what we know but still holds immense relevance. Looking backwards, we see a roadmap for advancing forward, towards a more holistic understanding of fitness that embraces mind and body as unified parts of the whole.

In our following chapters, we will dive deeper into the nutrition wisdom of these ancient cultures and see how they used the gifts of nature to fuel their bodies. Stay tuned to fortify your life with a dash of ancient wisdom, married beautifully with modern science.

Chapter 5. Primitive Diets: A Deeper Exploration

In the journey to understanding our ancestry and its nuanced implications on our present health, nothing proves as enchanting, or as enlightening, as the study of primitive diets.

Paradoxically, our technologically saturated modern lifestyles have bred a burgeoning interest in the simpler, more organic ways of our remote past. We seem to recognize intuitively the insidious health consequences of veering too far from the lifestyle to which evolution designed us. Recent studies confirm the prevailing suspicion that our prehistoric forebears, despite the hardship of their grueling existence, suffered significantly less from the so-called "diseases of civilization" that plague our era. Hence, going back to decode the principles of our predecessors' diets could partially illuminate our current health conundrums.

5.1. The Age of Hunters and Gatherers

About 2.6 million years ago, primordial humans began honing a critical survival skill that would undoubtedly influence the trajectory of civilization – hunting. As the epochs passed, our ancestors diversified their dietary tapestry, incorporating an assortment of plant foods as they gradually metamorphosized into efficient gatherers. This period, fondly known as the Paleolithic Era or the Age of Hunters and Gatherers, pens the maiden chapter in our rich dietary history.

Subsistence during this phase was largely dependent on wild, naturally grown foods. Our ancestors' meals were replete with lean meats, fish, fruits, vegetables, roots, and nuts - a stark contrast to the grain and processed food-laden diets of today. Fascinatingly, the dietary habits of modern-day primitive tribes, such as the Hazdas of Tanzania or the Amazonian Yanomami, who live bereft of agricultural or industrial influence, mirror this ancient genre of nutrition.

5.2. Nutritional Composition of Hunter-Gatherer Diets

Estimating the daily nutrient consumption of our Paleolithic predecessors is a formidable challenge, given the scant fossil record. However, anthropological explorations suggest a rough blueprint of their potential diet. The following narrative leans heavily on the work of Dr. Loren Cordain, one of the pioneers of Paleolithic nutrition studies.

Predominantly, the hunter-gatherer diet was low in saturated fats and entirely devoid of trans fats. Sodium was scarcer, with intakes substantially lower than we see in modern diets. Simultaneously, thanks to a bounty of fruits, vegetables, and lean meats, the Paleolithic meal plan was comparatively high in vitamins, minerals, unsaturated fats, and dietary fiber.

5.3. Comparisons with Modern Diets

Modern agricultural strides have certainly bulked up the variety and volume of edible fare we have access to. Still, they seem to have unexpectedly tinkered with the quality of our nutrition. The proliferation of processed, nutrient-deficient snacks, the widespread use of preservatives, and an abundance of omega-6 fatty acids (in lieu of the healthier omega-3 variants) stand as reproachful reminders of the detours we've taken from our initial dietary path.

It's all too easy to conclude that the key to good health is a return to a simple, Paleolithic-style diet. However, it's essential to remember that our physiological responses to a nutrient-intense, minimally processed diet have been established over thousands of years of evolutionary scrutiny. We might be, in reality, more adapted to these so-called 'primitive' diets than the grain-intensive, synthetic diets that we currently consume.

5.4. Health Implications of Primitive Diets

Unraveling the role of diet in our evolutionary past allows us to progressively realign our present nutrition - a practice that could potentially combat the rampant rise of non-communicable diseases. Studies indicate that a shift towards more primitive dietary practices, such as upping vegetable and fruit intake while diminishing processed food consumption, can remarkably improve several health measures.

Overall, the diet of our ancestors was not just about the foods they consumed but revolved around acquiring and appreciating natural, nutrient-dense sustenance. More than just a diet, it was a way of living harmoniously with the environment, a virtue we seem to have strayed from. It's on us, now, to retrace these lost connections, to rediscover the wisdom engraved in our evolutionary roots, and to slowly chart a healthier culinary course for our future.

Chapter 6. The Art of Fasting: Lessons from the Ancients

Long before the terms 'ketosis', 'intermittent fasting', or the trendier 'biohacking', our ancestors applied what we would now call fasting for survival, spiritual pursuits, and wellness. From the stone-age hunter rapt in the pursuit of his next meal, to the stoic philosopher advocating self-restraint, to the austere yogi meditating on the peaks of the Himalayas, the practice of deliberate abstention from food has echoed across ages and cultures.

6.1. Pioneers Of Fasting: The Hunter-Gatherers

Around two million years ago, the advent of the homo habilis marked a crucial juncture in our evolutionary journey. These early human ancestors were not just gatherers; they took a revolutionary leap onto the hunting grounds. These early hunters had a necessarily intermittent feeding pattern - they ate when they made their kill and fasted in between. The human body, splendid in its adaptability, responded to this eat-fast pattern by developing mechanisms to store surplus energy intake as fat for use during lean periods. This formed the basis for our capacity to fast without significant harm.

A review of our ancestral dietary patterns underscores the power and potential of the human body for endurance and adaptability, concepts that are fundamental to unlock the art of fasting.

6.2. Fasting in Antiquity: Philosophy and Religion

Fast-forward to the cradle of civilization, and one discovers fasting entwined with the cultural, religious and philosophical fabrics of ancient societies.

In ancient Greece, the legendary Pythagoras famously fasted for 40 days, believing that it sharpened his mind and promoted clear thinking. He required his students to fast before attending his lectures. Even the father of medicine, Hippocrates, advocated fasting, stating that: "To eat when you are sick, is to feed your illness."

In the East, the Vedic culture revered the practice of 'Upavasa' (fasting). Buddhist monks observed 'Vara', fasting from noon to the next morning. Many Biblical figures, including Moses, Jesus, and Elijah, undertook prolonged periods of fast.

These historical anecdotes emphasize fasting as a tool beyond physical health. Fasting was integral to mental clarity, spiritual growth, and even moral fortitude.

6.3. Delving into Biology: Understanding Ketosis

Now, let's delve into the biological underpinnings of fasting. When we fast, the body undergoes profound metabolic changes. After the depletion of dietary glucose, the reserve glycogen in the liver is utilized. Within 12-72 hours of fasting, the body enters into a state of 'ketosis' - a process in which the liver converts stored fats into 'ketone bodies'.

Ketone bodies act as an alternative fuel to glucose. They reduce oxidative stress and enhance the production of brain-derived neurotropic factors (BDNF), boosting cognitive functions and promoting overall health.

6.4. Adopting Ancient Wisdom: Intermittent Fasting

The echoes of the ancient fasting wisdom can be heard in the modern practice of 'Intermittent Fasting' (IF). It is a term for an eating pattern that cycles between periods of eating and fasting. The popular 16/8 method (16 hours of fasting and 8 hours of eating) is one such example that rekindles our hunter-gatherer roots.

What's interesting is the range of benefits that emerge from intermittent fasting. From weight loss, improved markers of health decreased inflammation, enhanced brain health to potential cancer prevention - the list goes on.

Decades of scientific research and a number of studies have now reinforced what our ancestors intuitively knew about fasting.

6.5. The Future of Fasting: Prescriptive Periods without Food

As we continue to appreciate the essence of fasting, we are branching into newer methodologies, like the 5:2 diet (eating normally for five days and eating less for two days in a week).

Yet the future journey is about more than devising newer fasting methods. It will entail understanding the nuances - the best practices for fasts, personalized timings based on one's genetic makeup, and determining the cases where fasting could be detrimental. It's about harking back to ancient wisdom while embracing the advances of modern science.

Fasting, as a millennia-old principle, is indeed an art. It is undeniably a testament to the enduring wisdom of our ancestors and their understanding of the human body. Its relevance in the present is potent, with the potential to shape a healthier future, both for the individual and mankind at large. As we teeter on the brink of remarkable scientific discoveries, it is indeed time to embrace the past to enhance our present, and ultimately, our future, in the timeless story of human health and wellbeing.

Chapter 7. The Ancient Practice of Meditation for Mind and Body Wellness

Meditation – this ancient practice, known to humans since the dawn of recorded history, has quietly stood the test of time, surpassing any passing trend. Its endurance and surging modern day relevance suggests its profound impact upon human wellness. The journey into the ancient practices of meditation organically weaves through an understanding of its cultural roots, the importance of the mind-body connection, meditative techniques, and the science grounding its usefulness.

7.1. Origins, Landscapes and Cultural Roots

Meditation as a practice emerged from the lands of ancient India, traced back 5000-3500 BCE, as per pictographic evidence. It was an integral part of Vedic Hindu culture, serving as a tool to train the mind and consciousness. The practice transcended borders and breezed across cultures; in Taoist China and Buddhist India around the 6th to the 5th centuries BCE, meditation emerged as a fundamental spiritual practice. The West began to embrace meditation much later, with the advent of Transcendental Meditation in the mid-twentieth century.

7.2. Mind-Body Connection

Meditation's power lies at the heart of the intriguing nexus between the mind and body. The harmony and interplay between these two elements of our existence set the stage for our overall wellbeing. Our thoughts, feelings, and mental states can influence physiological functioning, and an understanding of this intricate relationship underpins the practice of meditation. Through meditation, one can experience increased self-awareness and focus, which subsequently helps manage stress, anxiety and induce the state of relaxation.

7.3. Meditation Techniques

Meditation encompasses a spectrum of practices, each with roots dipping into various traditions and paths to enhance wellness.

1. Mindfulness Meditation: Rooted in Buddhist traditions, this practice encourages mindful awareness of the present moment. It gently nudges away distractions and disperses rumination, guiding towards a serene acceptance of the present.

2. Transcendental Meditation: This involves the repetition of a specific sound or mantra, practiced for 15-20 minutes twice daily. This method advocates the journey from the frenetic surface of thoughts down to the calm deep of consciousness.

3. Body Scan or Progressive Relaxation: This technique prompts to scan your body for areas of stress. The goal here is not merely to acknowledge stress, but to allow it to dissolve.

4. Breath Awareness Meditation: A type of mindful meditation that encourages mindful breathing. It boosts concentration by asking practitioners to focus on their breath.

5. Loving-Kindness Meditation: The goal here is to generate feelings of compassion and love, first for oneself and subsequently for others. It intends to foster an attitude of love and kindness towards everything, even sources of stress.

7.4. The Science Behind Meditation

Modern science is gradually unfolding and corroborating what the ancients had intuitively known about meditation. A multitude of research studies reveal its numerous benefits, intricately linking the practice with physical, psychological, and cognitive health. Meditation helps to decrease inflammation at the cellular level, reduce stress and anxiety, improve sleep, increase pain tolerance, boost immunity, and enhance focus and memory.

Advancements in neuroimaging techniques have facilitated a peek into the meditating brain, revealing structural changes, increased cortical thickness, decreased amygdala reactivity, and improved connectivity between various brain regions. Reduced symptoms of depression and anxiety align with these observed physiological changes, suggesting that our minds really can influence our bodies.

7.5. Conclusion: The Past Connects with the Present

Despite its age-old roots, meditation remains relevant today because it addresses the universal human need for peace, balance, and wellness. The ancient practice provides potent tools to nurture our minds and bodies amidst the unhindered hustle of modern life. By embracing this wisdom from the yore, we can navigate our way towards improved wellbeing, setting the stage for enhanced longevity and quality of life.

Through the course of this journey, it becomes increasingly evident that ancient practices, like meditation, intertwined with adaptations for the current lifestyle, can truly optimize wellness. As we continue to unravel the wisdom our ancestors left behind, the path towards health and happiness becomes clear and increasingly within reach.

Chapter 8. Herbs and Superfoods: The Forgotten Nutritional Staples

Long before advancements in modern technique and nutritional science, our ancestors had an intuitive grasp of the powers imbued in nature. This knowledge was passed down through generations, with traditional medicine often utilizing herbs and what we now call 'superfoods' due to their abundant nutritional value. For them, these were the mainstays that optimized health and vitality. Yet, in our quest for quick fixes and the allure of sophisticated nutritional strategies, these unassuming staples have been inadvertently forgotten.

8.1. The Umbral Potency of Herbs

Herbs have been a staple part of the human diet and holistic medicine for thousands of years. In the context of nutrition, they offer an impressive array of vitamins, minerals, fibers, antioxidants, and a multitude of other disease-fighting compounds.

A classic example is the use of garlic—prized in ancient societies for its medical properties—research now confirms its versatile benefits such as immune support, cancer prevention, and heart health. The active compound allicin, released when garlic is crushed or chewed, is a potent therapeutic agent responsible for most of its impressive health benefits.

Similarly, turmeric, well-known in Indian traditional medicine (Ayurveda), is another excellent example. The active compound, curcumin, possesses potent anti-inflammatory and antioxidant effects that have been thoroughly studied by modern science.

Herbs like cilantro, parsley, and dill not only pack intense flavors but are also rich in antioxidants and vitamins, making them worth the extra sprinkle on your dishes. Cultivating a habit of including versatile herbs like basil, mint, rosemary, and thyme in your cooking can not only enhance the taste but significantly uplift the nutritional profile of your meals.

In essence, integrating these herbs into your daily dietary regime allows you to harness the manifold health benefits they offer—from enhanced digestion to improved immune function and beyond.

8.2. Rediscovering the Classics: Superfoods

In recent times, the term "superfoods" has become something of a buzzword. Defined as nutrient-rich food considered beneficial to health and well-being, superfoods have been marketed heavily due to their perceived health benefits. However, it's interesting to note that these superfoods have deep roots in ancient, traditional diets.

Quinoa, a seed initially discovered in the Andes of South America, was a staple food for the ancient Incas, who referred to it as 'the mother of all grains'. Now recognized as a superfood globally, it offers a perfect balance of all nine essential amino acids for humans, making it an excellent source of plant-based protein. Also, quinoa is rich in fiber, magnesium, B vitamins, iron, potassium, calcium, phosphorus, vitamin E, and various beneficial antioxidants.

Similarly, berries, rich in immune-boosting antioxidants and vitamins, have been a part of indigenous diets for centuries. The elderberry, for example, has been used for its immune-boosting properties, while blueberries have been linked to enhancing brain health.

Spinach, while a common leafy green, is a powerhouse of nutrients.

Rich in vitamins A, C, K and minerals like magnesium and iron, it's an excellent boost for overall health.

Studies have even found that almonds, initially cultivated in Iran and surrounding countries, were medicinal and nutritional powerhouses in several ancient civilizations. Loaded with antioxidants, high amounts of heart-healthy monounsaturated fats, and fiber, they are a wholesome snack that can curb hunger and provide substantial nutrition.

Incorporating these superfoods into your diet reinforces your body with an arsenal of beneficial nutrients designed to foster optimal health and well-being.

8.3. Balancing Flavors and Nutrients

Understanding how to meld the forceful flavors of herbs and the powerhouse nutritional profiles of superfoods into one's diet requires knowledge and practice. Adding too many robust herbs can overpower a meal, while a steady diet of superfood salads may become monotonous.

Balancing these elements begins with trial and error. Start with familiar recipes and gradually introduce new herbs or superfoods. Make a simple quinoa salad with fresh herbs, or switch your white rice with nutrient-rich brown rice or farro. Experiment with using turmeric or ginger in your tea, or add a refreshing mix of berries to your breakfast cereal or smoothie.

Over time, these small changes can turn into habits, and you'll find your meals not only taste better but are more satisfying and nutritious.\n === Concluding Thoughts

Herbs and superfoods are not merely present-day fad or marketing buzzwords but have firm roots in ancestral nutrition practices. In their unassuming ways, they tether us to the land and our history, providing us rich, dense nutrition. Utilizing them allows us to connect with our roots and honor age-old traditions while setting the foundation for a healthier present and future.

In essence, rediscovering and re-incorporating these overlooked nutritional staples is a wholesome approach to elevate our health and wellness. It's a gentle reminder that sometimes the answers to our modern problems lie embedded in the wisdom of the past.

Chapter 9. Traditional Healing Methods and Their Modern Implications

Historically, humankind has demonstrated an inherent reliance on natural elements and traditional rituals for health and healing. Long before laboratories synthetized medications, our ancestors turned to the earth to find remedies for a plethora of maladies. Today, in our technologically-powered world, it has become imperative to rekindle that lost connection with traditional healing methods, recognizing their value and understanding their modern implications.

9.1. The Dawn of Healing Traditions

The story of traditional healing methods has its roots in the cradle of civilization. The earliest human societies turned to their immediate surroundings to deal with injuries, diseases, and ailments. These early healing practices often involved the use of medicinal plants, massage, spiritual rituals, and mind-body exercises.

Primordial peoples developed a deep respect for the power of the earth's bounty. They meticulously observed, catalogued, and experimented with various plants, attributing healing properties to many. Herbal remedies became a cornerstone of their healing practices.

They also understood the importance of physical touch and movement, leading to the development of early forms of massage and exercise routines. With a profound sense of spirituality, they performed rituals and ceremonies to banish ill health and protect against perceived malevolent forces.

This magic merge of the physical, natural, and spiritual formed the foundation of our ancestors' healing traditions, many of which continue to be relevant today.

9.2. Traditional Remedies: Rediscovering Herbal Medicine

Traditional herbal medicine amplifies the notion of 'Nature as Healer.' The sheer volume of medicinal plants available to our ancestors resulted in an exhaustive pharmacopoeia of herbal treatments.

Modern science has validated many of these. For instance, willow bark used by ancient Egyptians for pain and inflammation offered us aspirin. Cinchona bark used by South American tribes to combat malaria led to the extraction of quinine.

These are just the tip of the iceberg. There's a chest of potent natural remedies waiting to be rediscovered, reinterpreted, and embedded in our modern pharmacology.

9.3. Going Hands-On: The Therapeutic Power of Touch

The power of touch has been esteemed for millennia. Traditional arts like massage, acupressure, and chiropractic techniques exemplify this. By manipulating muscles, applying pressure to specific points, or aligning the spine, our ancestors promoted circulation, relieved pain, improved mobility, and more.

Today, methods like massage and physiotherapy still use the fundamental concepts of touch therapy. As mental health gains more attention, the calming effect of human touch is being recognized to treat trauma, stress, and anxiety.

9.4. Spiritual Healing: Modern Views on Ancient Rituals

In ancient cultures, spiritual practices often played a role in healing. Shamans, medicine men, and healers were revered, their rituals bringing together communities and manifesting collective will to banish disease.

While many of these approaches might seem archaic today, we can still extract valuable lessons. Modern practices such as meditation, mindfulness, and some aspects of psychotherapy owe much to the spiritual wisdom of our forebears.

9.5. The Ancient Art of Staying Active

The health benefits of physical activity were not lost on our ancestors. From early forms of yoga in the East to Roman strength training in the West, keeping active was integral to their lifestyle, contributing to overall health.

Modern fitness regimens have evolved significantly but still exhibit ancestral echoes. Today's strength and conditioning, flexibility workouts, and cardiovascular drills bear ancient imprints. We now have research affirming what our ancestors intuitively understood – that regular exercise is a potent antidote to many of today's leading health issues.

Rediscovering and applying these traditional healing methods doesn't entail denying modern medical advancements. It is about forging a complementary path in our pursuit of wellness, amalgamating the best of the old and the new, and creating an unhindered, holistic healing environment. By perusing our past with curiosity and openness, we illuminate our present with newfound wisdom and practical tools to better manage our health.

Chapter 10. Adapting Ancient Wisdom to Modern Lifestyle

The dawn of mankind witnessed an instinctual alignment with nature, and our ancestors discovered countless gems of wisdom through their practised observation of natural systems and phenomena. These fundamental insights formed the basis of their food habits, physical exercises, and lifestyle patterns, ensuring their robust health and longevity. Today, however, as we grapple with challenges of an artificial, sedentary lifestyle, it becomes pertinently essential to revisit these roots, to adapt the ancient wisdom to our modern lifestyle.

10.1. Tapping into Ancestral Diets

Unprocessed foods, whole grains, fruits, and vegetables were the mainstays of our ancestors' diet, providing vital macro and micro-nutrients necessary for optimal health. Today, in our fast-paced lives, we often rely heavily on processed foods. However, a shift towards more natural and whole foods, heralding an era of 'clean eating,' mimics the purity and nutritional wealth of ancestral diets.

Include more seasonal and locally grown food in your meals. The ancients believed that food comprises more than mere calories; they treated it as a therapeutic modality. Ignore the fads offering quick fixes and instead heed to the ancient practice of balanced and mindful eating.

Tips for Incorporating Whole Foods into Your Daily Diet

- Begin with simple swaps, such as replacing white bread and pasta with whole grain alternatives.

- Snack on a mix of seasonal fruits, nuts, and seeds instead of processed snacks.

- Incorporate legumes, lentils, green leafy vegetables in your daily meals.

- Sip on homemade herbal teas and infusions instead of sugar-laden drinks.

- Redefine 'fast food' with quick and easy homemade meals.

10.2. Reclaiming Physical Activity

The essence of ancient physical practices lay in the holistic development of the body, and not solely in muscular growth. Our ancestors incorporated movements that enhanced strength, flexibility, endurance, and balance. From the flowing postures of Yoga to the discipline of martial arts, these practices were not just exercises but philosophies implemented to enhance every facet of life.

Creating an exercise routine that aligns with these principles can significantly improve your fitness profile. Incorporate various forms of exercises such as resistance training, Yoga, Pilates, or even simple activities like dancing and hiking.

10.3. The Art of Mindful Presence

The ancients deeply understood the symbiotic relationship between the mind, body, and nature. They practiced mindfulness not as a separate activity, but as an integral part of their lives. In modern times, we could benefit from inculcating this practice into our everyday routines. Focus on one task at a time, savor your meals, and take time to appreciate the simple joys of life.

Attempting to digitize mindfulness into apps can prove counterproductive as the very act of mindfulness requires us to detach from our digital devices. Instead, practice simple breathing exercises, meditation, and adequate sleep, about 7-9 hours for adults, as these are essential for mental tranquility and enhancing cognitive functions.

10.4. The Science of Nature's Healing Power

Our ancestors had a profound understanding of the curative properties of plants, and many remedies developed by them have withstood the test of time. In our modern world, which is inhabited by new-age diseases, these remedies can provide natural alternatives to chemical medications.

An enriched understanding of these plant-based remedies and their appropriate usage can facilitate better health and wellbeing. For instance, the routine use of spices like turmeric, cinnamon, and ginger in our meals can bolster our immunity and fend off various ailments. Respect nature's pharmacy, but exercise caution and moderation in usage. Ensure to consult with modern healthcare providers before substituting any prescribed medication.

In summary, adapting ancient wisdom entails making informed choices about our diet, improving exercise regimens, developing mindfulness, and utilizing nature's healing prowess. By combining elements of traditional practices with modern understanding, we can navigate towards healthier, more fulfilling lives. Remember, adapting doesn't mean eradicating modern conveniences; it means refining our lifestyles to embody the best from the old and the new. This, in essence, would be our Legacy Lifestyle – an all-encompassing lifestyle that honors the past, empowers the present, and preserves the future.

Chapter 11. The Future of Fitness and Nutrition: Bridging the Past and the Present

As we move forward, steeped in a flurry of scientific discoveries and technological advancements, we must pause and recognize the value of our heritage. The wisdom inherent in the fitness and nutrition practices of our ancestors can guide our contemporary pursuit of wellness and health. This chapter aims to explore this fascinating intersection, bridging the gap between the past and the present, and postulating a future where time-tried traditions significantly inform our present and future wellness strategies.

11.1. Historical Fitness and Nutrition Practices

The primitive understanding of fitness was a far cry from what we associate with it today. For our ancestors, fitness was a means of survival - whether hunting for prey, evading predators, or traversing vast landscapes. Similarly, their approach to nutrition had less to do with counting calories and more with deriving sustenance to support the physical exertion their lives necessitated.

Interestingly, this functional approach to fitness and nutrition highlights a key lesson: the alignments between body function, physical activity, and food intake reach far beyond mere calorie counting towards preserving overall body health and promoting longevity.

11.2. Modern Science and Ancestral Wisdom: A Confluence

Modern research is progressively supporting many traditional fitness and nutrition practices. Scientists are discovering that intermittent fasting, a practice reminiscent of the feast and famine cycles experienced by our ancestors, could have several health benefits. This includes weight loss, improved markers of health, and a reduced risk of chronic diseases.

Similarly, traditional physical activities, often routinized into daily life (like farming, foraging, or walking long distances), are being validated for their comprehensive impacts on cardiovascular health and muscle-building.

11.3. The Optimization of Traditional Practices

The goal isn't to revert entirely to ancestral lifestyles. Instead, we aim to incorporate lessons from the past into our contemporary lives, to create an optimized version of fitness and nutrition fit for the modern individual.

For instance, an application of our ancestral propensity for motion involves incorporating more 'natural movements' into our workout routines. This could include variations of walking, running, jumping, crawling, and balancing that closely mimic the full-body, functional movements our ancestors would have utilized.

Nutrition-wise, the lesson from the past can be seen in appreciating the simplicity and wholesomeness of foods. Ancient diets were devoid of processed items and replete with natural, whole foods— an approach mirrored in modern nutrition philosophies like the 'clean eating' movement or 'paleo diet'.

11.4. Technological Innovations and Ancestral Interventions

Technology has the potential to play a critical role in personalizing and enhancing these ancient wisdoms. Mobile applications can introduce traditional fitness routines within the convenience of our homes. Wearable technology can provide real-time feedback on intensity and form, ensuring that these traditional exercises are performed effectively and safely.

Nutrition apps can provide us with personalized dietary recommendations based on our unique genetics, microbiome, and lifestyle needs. These apps can track our food intake and provide guidance for achieving an optimal nutritional balance. In the future, we may even see AI-driven platforms that can recommend personalized meal plans based on our genetic predispositions – bringing the wisdom of our genetic ancestry to our dinner tables.

11.5. The Future: A Call for Balance

The future of fitness and nutrition lies in a balance— a balance between the simplicity of ancestral lifestyles and the complexities of modern life. New discoveries on the horizon, like gene editing or nanotechnology, promise to further revolutionize our understanding of fitness and nutrition. Yet, as we look towards this horizon, we would do well to remember the lessons from our past.

In summary, the integration of historical wisdom and modern understanding is more than a nostalgic nod to our human history. It is a robust roadmap for our future health and wellbeing. By blending time-honored traditions with modern research and technological innovations, we can create a comprehensive, personalized approach to fitness and nutrition that isn't just about living longer, but living better.